Keto Diet Cookbook With Poultry

Delicious Ketogenic Poultry Recipes for Your Diet

I0145889

By

Elisa Hayes

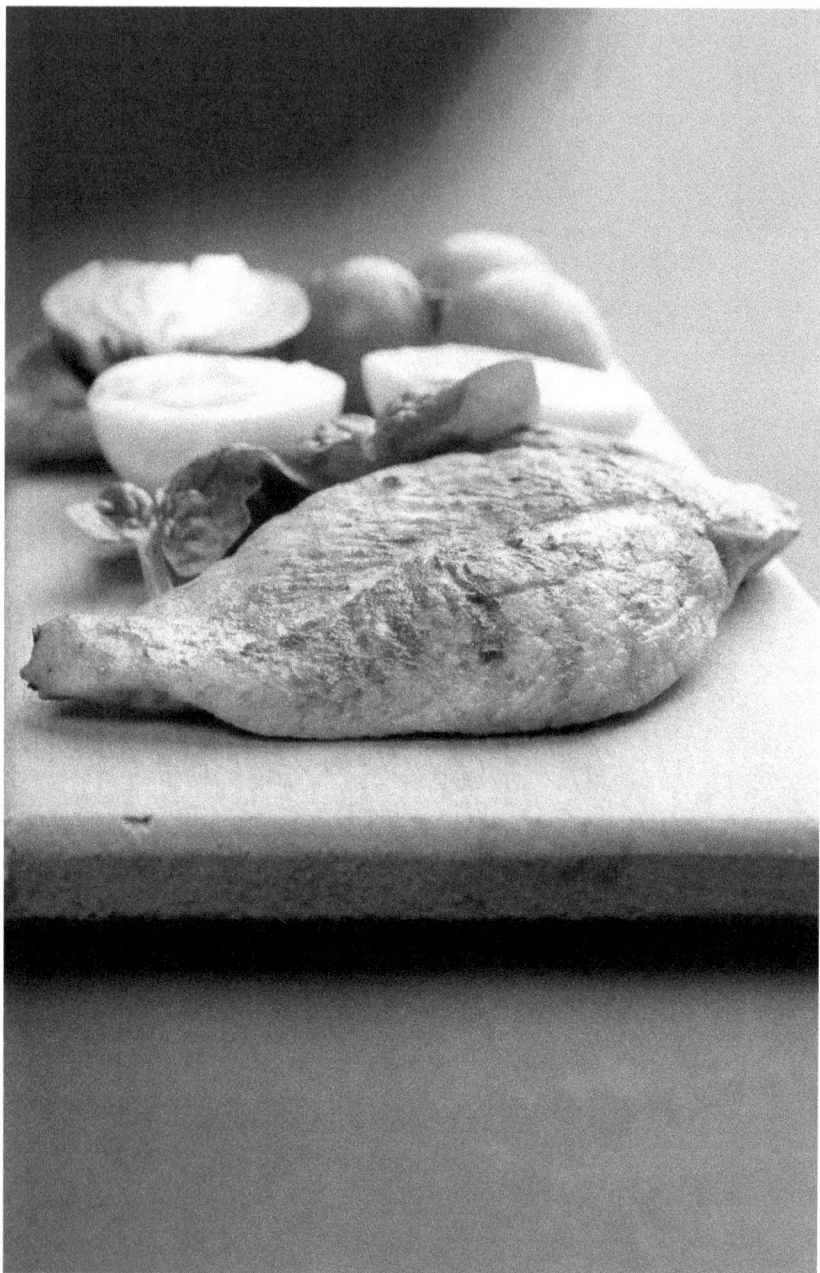

Table of Contents

The information in the following pages is broadly considered a truthful and accurate account of facts and as such, any inattention, use, or misuse of the information in question by the reader will render any resulting actions solely under their purview. There are no scenarios in which the publisher or the original author of this work can be in any fashion deemed liable for any hardship or damages that may befall them after undertaking information described herein.

Additionally, the information in the following pages is intended only for informational purposes and should thus be thought of as universal. As befitting its nature, it is presented without assurance regarding its prolonged validity or interim quality. Trademarks that are mentioned are done without written consent and can in no way be considered an endorsement from the trademark holder.

Introduction

The path to a perfect body and good physical health was very thorny for me. The only one wish which I was making for my birthdays for many years was to be a slim and beautiful girl. Alas, everything can't be as in fairy tales and the miracle didn't happen; my mirror was still showing the same fat, pimple girl. In childhood, the problem of being overweight didn't bother me much; I can say that I didn't care about it at all, I didn't know that weight would be momentous for me. I was an ordinary smiling child, playing with my peers, going to school, and traveling with my parents. That time my chubby cheeks seemed very sweet to everyone. But that was then. At 11-year-old, I went to middle school. New people, new teachers, I had no friends at all. Mentally I was broken. I counted the minutes until the end of the last lesson, to quickly sit in my mom's car and leave school. I started to eat a lot. Now I see that in this way I am stressed, but then the food served as my antidepressant. Dozens of hamburgers, fried potatoes, coke – they were "my best friends". In addition to everything, I started to have horrible skin problems, it seemed to me that there was no place on my face wherever they hadn't appeared yet. Time passed and I no longer loved my reflection in the mirror even in 1%. I couldn't wear the clothes that I liked. I usually wore oversized shorts and t-shirts. I couldn't afford to wear a short dress and high heels. At 15-year-old I weighed more than 270lbs. I remember what I felt in those days, as it is happening now. I felt anger, irritation, hatred, and self-loathing. That prom party was the most terrible day of my life. Thank God it's over!

In those years, the keto diet was not very popular, fasting and drinking diets (which, as you already know, did not help me much) were more popular. Perhaps I wouldn't do anything, but my health problems were becoming more serious. It seemed that my body was simply screaming: please help me!

I remember the day that changed my life on a dime. I came to the clinic with pain in my stomach. But this time, I not only received painkillers but also found a mentor and friend. This was my physician. She had examined me and recommended that I go on a diet. I didn't want to do something and was categorically against it. However, my mind changed when she said: love your body, care about it, and it will thank you. What was my surprise when the diet turned out to be very simple to follow. Is it so easy to love myself? As you could understand I am talking about my favorite keto diet. Every day I was eating a maximum of proteins and a minimum of carbohydrates. That meant to consume meat, poultry, and fish and make restrictions for vegetables, fruits, and sweets. After 2 weeks, I lost 83lbs, and further results were getting better and better. All this time I was under the supervision of a doctor and this yielded results. A year later, I completely changed all the clothes in my wardrobe and oh my God I was able to wear a short dress and skirts! Now I can say that I am the happiest person. It happened because I fell in love with myself and started treating my body as a diamond. My life was filled with bright colors, I have a beloved husband, children, work, friends, I am healthy and like myself in the mirror. I am telling this story to prove that the right diet can solve almost all problems with body and health. It is a fact that our body is capable of dealing with dramatic changes, it is only worth loving it. Never rest on your laurels, never give up and forbid people to say that you cannot do something. You are already a great fellow that you bought this cookbook and decided to take a step ahead in the direction to your dream. Let this book become your ray of hope, a lifesaver on the way to your wonderful transformation. If you believe in yourself and love your body, believe me, the result won't be long in coming. You will see in the mirror a completely new version of yourself, updated physically and mentally! Just trust the keto diet and your inner voice. Set a goal today and start the way of achieving it right now. Don't try to do it all in one time; let it be a small step day by day. Exactly now, this is the right time to start creating a new version of you. If this diet was able to change my life, I'm sure it will help you too!

Garlic Chicken

Prep time: 10 minutes

Cook time: 12 minutes

Servings: 2

Ingredients:

- ½ cup almond flour
- 1 egg, beaten
- 2 tablespoons minced garlic
- 2 chicken breasts, skinless, boneless, chopped
- 2 tablespoons coconut oil

Method:

1. Melt the coconut oil in the skillet.

2. Then mix chicken with minced garlic and egg.

3. After this, coat the chicken in the almond flour and put in the melted oil.

4. Roast the chicken for 5 minutes per side on the medium heat.

Nutritional info per serve: Calories 479, Fat 30.2, Fiber 0.9, Carbs 4.5, Protein 47

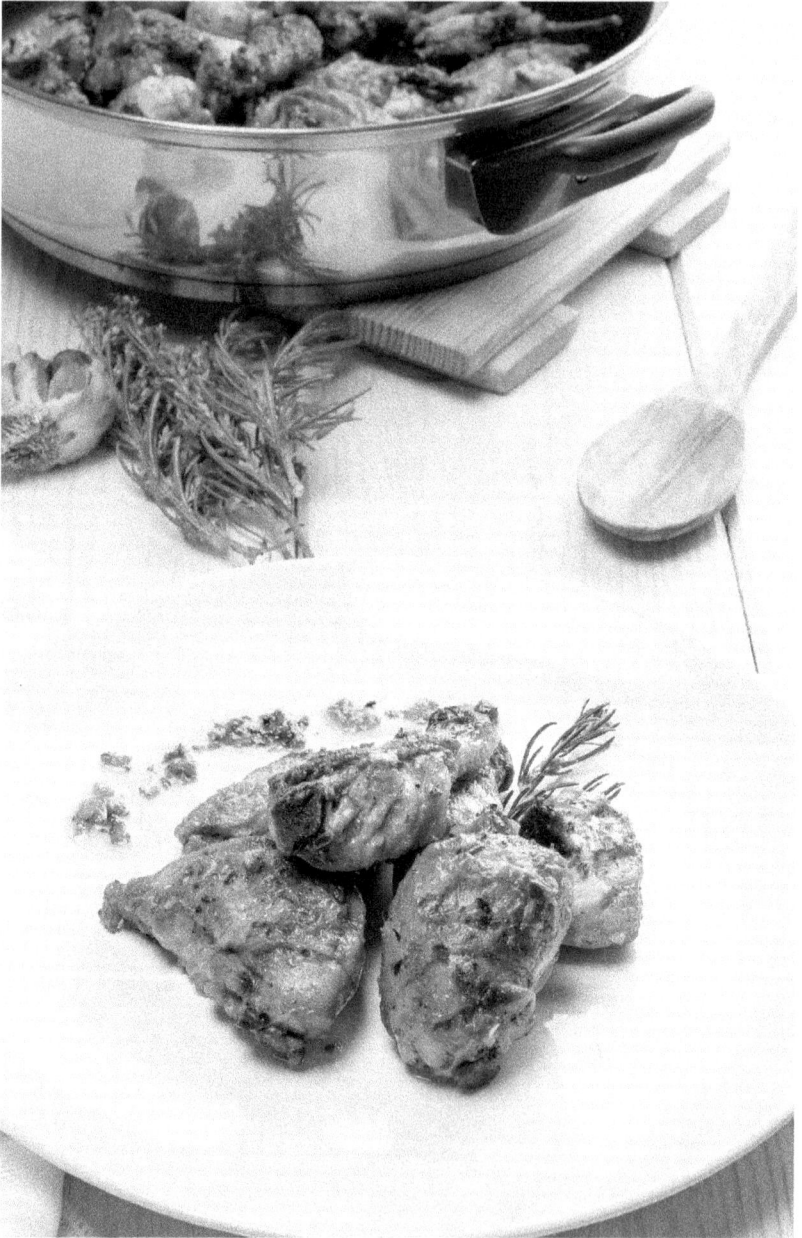

Chili Drumsticks

Prep time: 10 minutes

Cook time: 20 minutes

Servings:4

Ingredients:

- 4 chicken drumsticks
- 1 teaspoon chili flakes
- 1 teaspoon salt
- 1 teaspoon dried sage
- 1 tablespoon avocado oil

Method:

1. In the shallow bowl, mix chili flakes, salt, and dried sage.

2. Then mix chicken drumsticks with spice mixture.

3. After this, preheat the skillet well.

4. Put the chicken drumsticks in the skillet and roast the meal for 10 minutes per side on the medium heat.

Nutritional info per serve: Calories 83, Fat 3.1, Fiber 0.2, Carbs 0.3, Protein 12.7

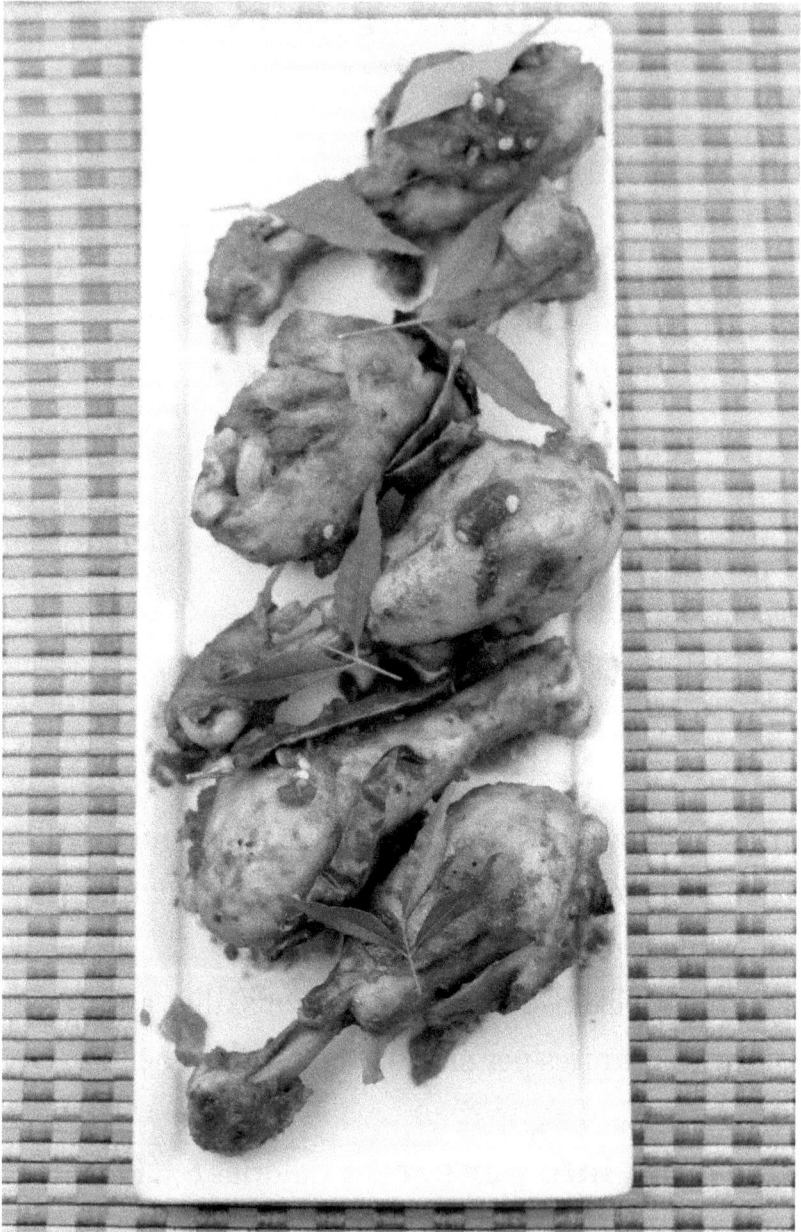

Sage Chicken Wings

Prep time: 10 minutes

Cook time: 30 minutes

Servings: 6

Ingredients:

- 1 teaspoon dried sage
- 1 teaspoon ground black pepper
- 6 chicken wings
- 1 tablespoon avocado oil

Method:

1. Mix the chicken wings with ground black pepper and dried sage.

2. Then sprinkle the chicken wings with avocado oil and transfer in the tray.

3. Bake the chicken wings for 30 minutes at 360F.

Nutritional info per serve: Calories 98, Fat 6.6, Fiber 0.3, Carbs 3.6, Protein 5.8

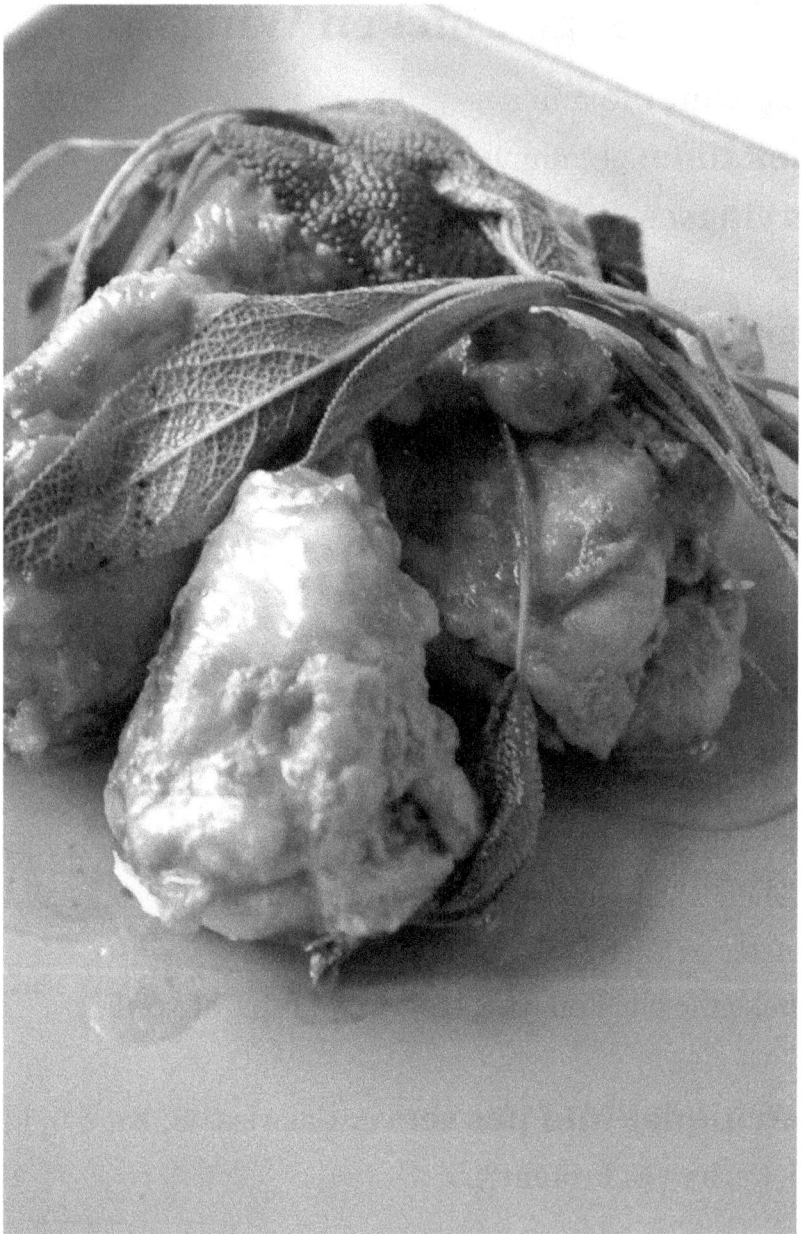

Oregano Chicken Wings

Prep time: 10 minutes

Cook time: 30 minutes

Servings:2

Ingredients:

- 4 chicken wings
- 1 tablespoon dried oregano
- 2 tablespoons avocado oil
- 1 tablespoon lemon juice

Method:

1. Sprinkle the chicken wings with dried oregano, avocado oil, and lemon juice.

2. Then put them in the baking tray and bake at 365F for 30 minutes. Flip the chicken wings on another side after 15 minutes of cooking.

Nutritional info per serve: Calories 345, Fat 23.4, Fiber 1.9, Carbs 13.1, Protein 20

Chicken Meatballs

Prep time: 10 minutes

Cook time: 10 minutes

Servings: 3

Ingredients:

- 1 teaspoon dried oregano
- 1 teaspoon chili powder
- 1 teaspoon dried cilantro
- 1 cup ground chicken
- 1 teaspoon coconut oil

Method:

1. In the mixing bowl, mix ground chicken, dried cilantro, chili powder, and dried oregano.

2. Then make the small meatballs.

3. Melt the coconut oil in the skillet.

4. Then put the chicken meatballs in the hot coconut oil and roast them for 4 minutes per side.

Nutritional info per serve: Calories 106, Fat 5.2, Fiber 0.5, Carbs 0.8, Protein 13.7

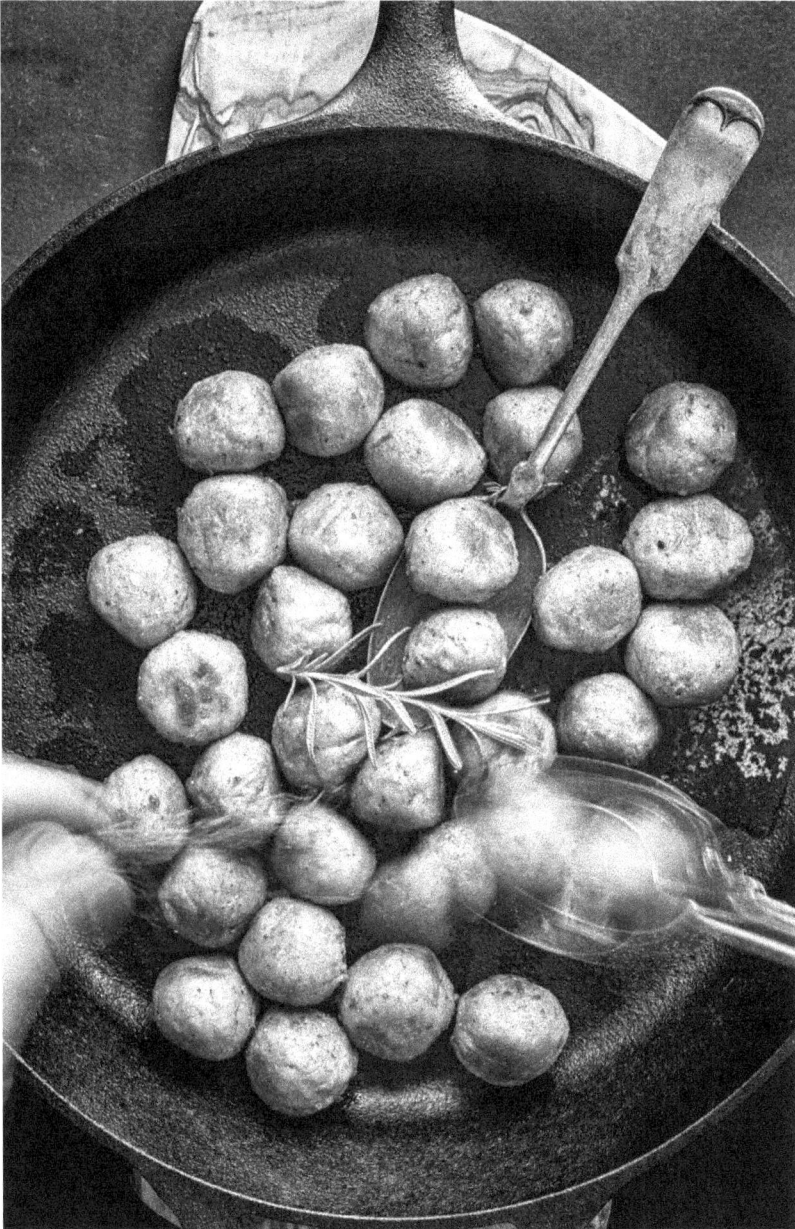

Paprika Chicken Wings

Prep time: 10 minutes

Cook time: 10 minutes

Servings:4

Ingredients:

- 10 oz chicken wings
- 1 tablespoon ground paprika
- 1 tablespoon avocado oil
- 1 teaspoon salt

Method:

1. Sprinkle the chicken wings with ground paprika and salt.

2. Then sprinkle the chicken ings with avocado oil and put in the hot skillet.

3. Roast the chicken wings for 4 minutes per side.

Nutritional info per serve: Calories 144, Fat 5.9, Fiber 0.8, Carbs 1.2, Protein 20.8

Lime Chicken Wings

Prep time: 10 minutes

Cook time: 10 minutes

Servings: 5

Ingredients:

- 5 chicken wings
- 1 teaspoon lime zest, grated
- 1 tablespoon avocado oil
- 3 tablespoons lime juice

Method:

1. Mix lime juice, avocado oil, and lime zest.

2. Then rub the chicken wings with avocado oil mixture.

3. Grill the chicken wings at 400F for 4 minutes.

Nutritional info per serve: Calories 99, Fat 6.7, Fiber 0.3, Carbs 3.8, Protein 5.8

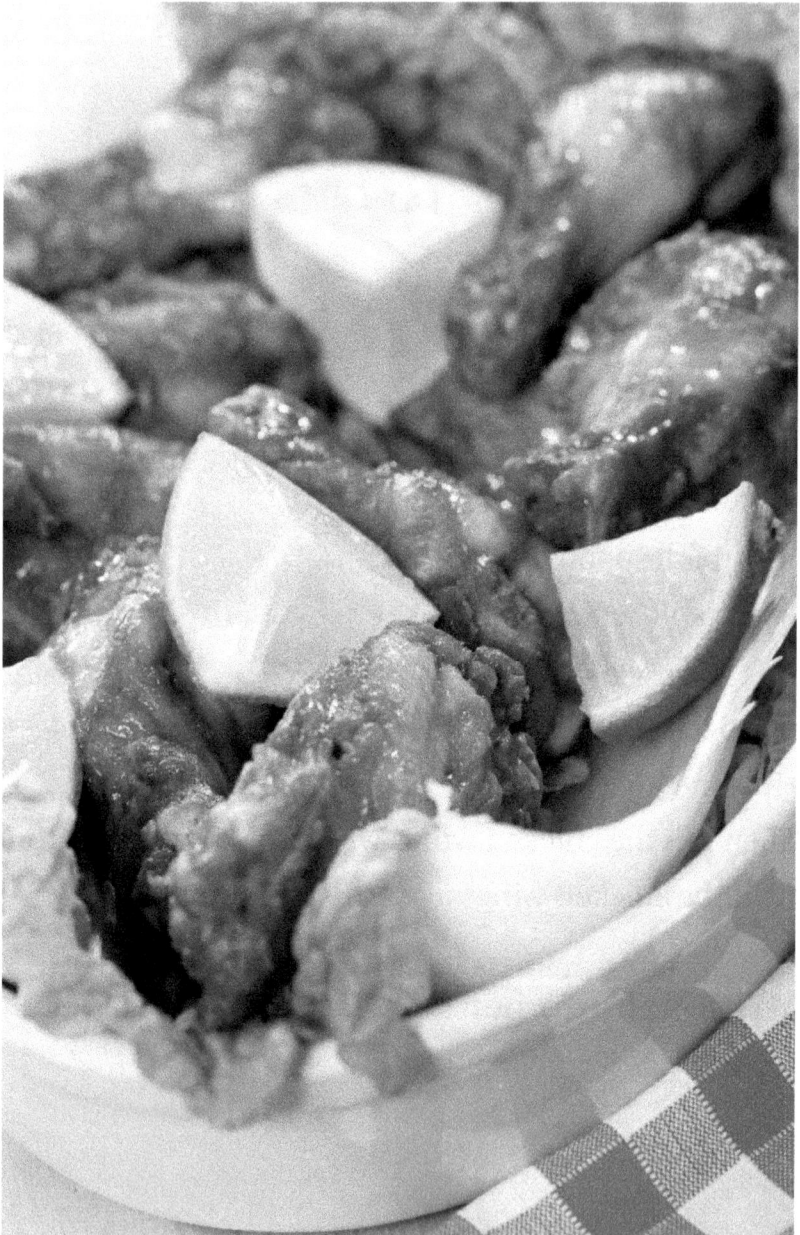

Coconut Chicken

Prep time: 10 minutes

Cook time: 20 minutes

Servings:6

Ingredients:

- 1-pound chicken breast, skinless, boneless, chopped
- ½ cup coconut cream
- 1 teaspoon dried oregano
- 1 teaspoon garlic powder
- ½ teaspoon ground paprika
- 1 tablespoon coconut oil

Method:

1. In the shallow bowl, mix ground paprika, garlic powder, and dried oregano.

2. Then mix the chicken breast with ground paprika mixture.

3. Then melt the coconut oil in the saucepan.

4. Add chicken and roast it for 4 minutes per side.

5. Add coconut cream and close the lid.

6. Cook the meal on medium heat for 10 minutes.

Nutritional info per serve: Calories 155, Fat 9, Fiber 0.7, Carbs 1.7, Protein 16.6

Onion Chicken

Prep time: 10 minutes

Cook time: 15 minutes

Servings: 4

Ingredients:

- 1-pound chicken fillet, sliced
- 2 spring onions, sliced
- 1 tablespoon coconut oil
- ½ teaspoon onion powder
- ½ teaspoon salt

Method:

1. Sprinkle the chicken fillet with spring onion powder and salt.

2. Then melt the coconut oil in the skillet.

3. Add onion and roast it for 5 minutes.

4. After this, stir the onion and add chicken fillet.

5. Roast the chicken with onion for 10 minutes on medium heat.

Nutritional info per serve: Calories 257, Fat 11.8, Fiber 0.6, Carbs 2.8, Protein 33.1

Almond Chicken

Prep time: 10 minutes

Cook time: 40 minutes

Servings:4

Ingredients:

- 11 oz chicken fillet
- 2 eggs, beaten
- ½ cup almond flour
- Cooking spray

Method:

1. Cut the chicken into 4 servings.

2. Then dip it in the eggs and coat in the almond flour.

3. Spray the baking tray with cooking spray and put the chicken inside.

4. Bake the chicken for 40 minutes at 355F.

Nutritional info per serve: Calories 200, Fat 9.7, Fiber 0.4, Carbs 0.9, Protein 26.1

Garlic and Dill Chicken

Prep time: 10 minutes

Cook time: 45 minutes

Servings: 4

Ingredients:

- 2 tablespoons avocado oil
- 1 teaspoon minced garlic
- 1 teaspoon dried dill
- 1-pound chicken breast, skinless, boneless

Method:

1. Mix dill with avocado oil and dried dill.

2. Then rub the chicken breast with avocado oil mixture and wrap in the foil.

3. Bake the chicken at 360F for 45 minutes.

Nutritional info per serve: Calories 140, Fat 3.7, Fiber 0.4, Carbs 0.8, Protein 24.2

Cheese Chicken Casserole

Prep time: 15 minutes

Cook time: 50 minutes

Servings:6

Ingredients:

- 1-pound chicken breast, skinless, boneless, chopped
- 1 cup Cheddar cheese, shredded
- 1 tablespoon butter, softened
- ½ teaspoon chili flakes
- ½ cup of water
- 1 cup bell pepper, chopped

Method:

1. Grease the casserole mold with butter.

2. Then mix chicken breast with chili flakes and put in the casserole mold in one layer.

3. Top it with bell pepper and water.

4. Then add Cheddar cheese and flatten it well.

5. Bake the casserole at 360F for 50 minutes.

Nutritional info per serve: Calories 185, Fat 10.1, Fiber 0.3, Carbs 1.8, Protein 20.9

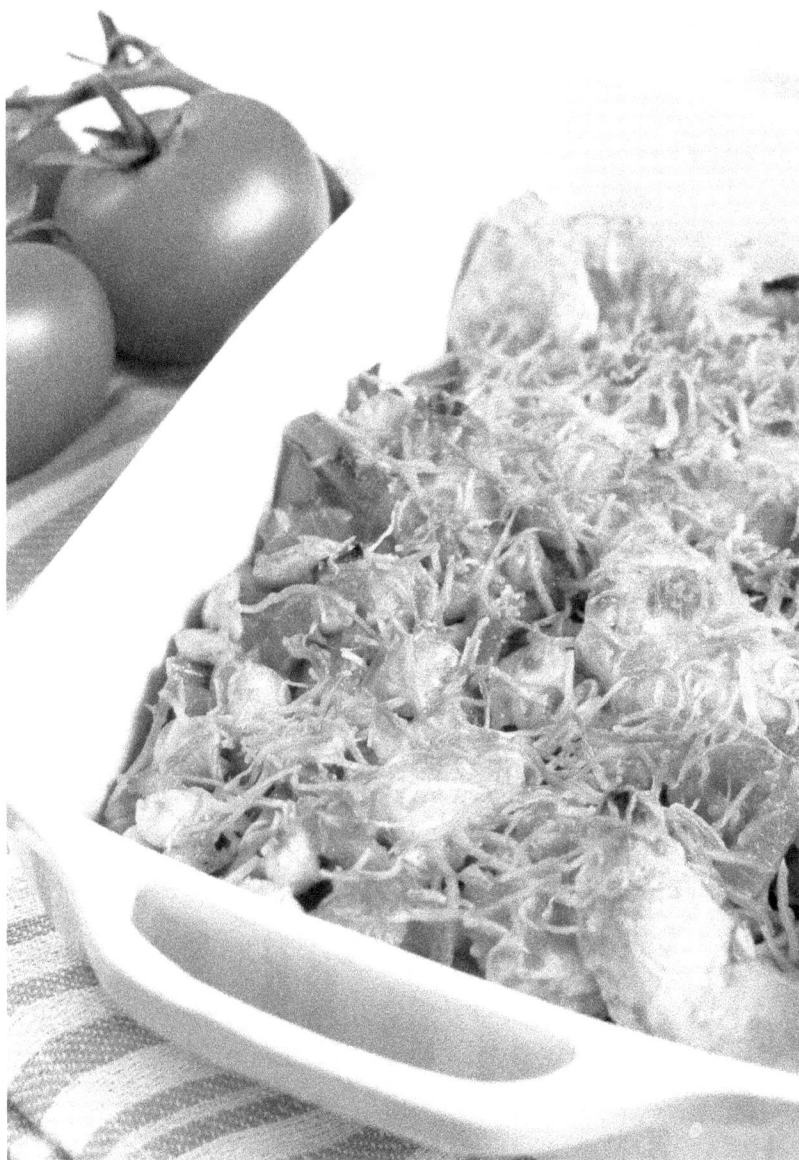

Lemon Chicken

Prep time: 10 minutes

Cook time: 40 minutes

Servings: 6

Ingredients:

- 6 chicken drumsticks
- ½ lemon, sliced
- 1 teaspoon salt
- 1 tablespoon butter

Method:

1. Grease the baking tray with butter.

2. Sprinkle the chicken drumsticks with salt and put it in the baking tray.

3. Top the chicken with sliced lemon and bake it for 40 minutes at 355F.

Nutritional info per serve: Calories 96, Fat 4.6, Fiber 0.1, Carbs 0.5, Protein 12.7

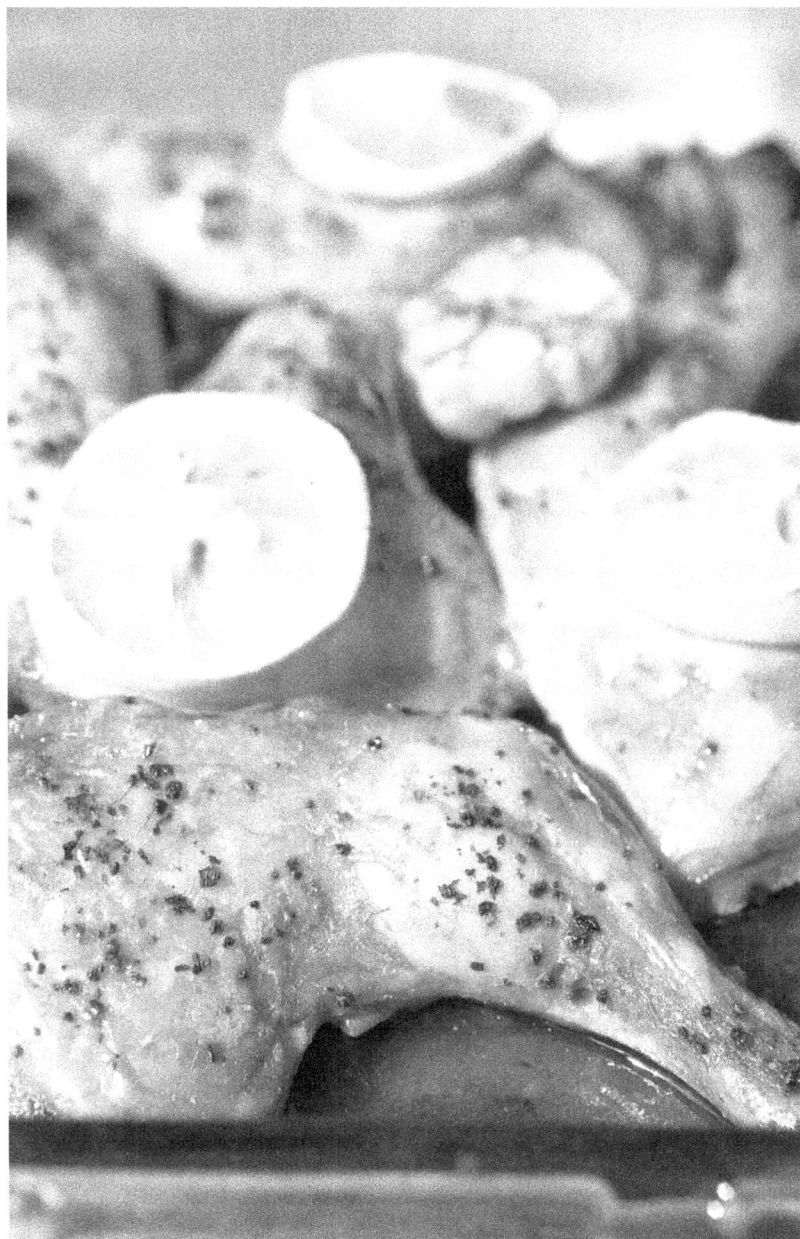

Italian Style Chicken

Prep time: 10 minutes

Cook time: 35 minutes

Servings:4

Ingredients:

- 4 chicken drumsticks
- 1 teaspoon dried oregano
- ½ teaspoon dried thyme
- 2 tablespoons avocado oil

Method:

1. Rub the chicken drumsticks with thyme and oregano.

2. Then sprinkle the chicken with avocado oil and put in the baking tray in one layer.

3. Bake the chicken at 360F for 35 minutes.

Nutritional info per serve: Calories 89, Fat 3.6, Fiber 0.5, Carbs 0.7, Protein 12.8

Paprika Chicken Fillet

Prep time: 10 minutes

Cook time: 10 minutes

Servings: 5

Ingredients:

- 1 tablespoon butter
- 1 teaspoon ground paprika
- ½ teaspoon ground turmeric
- 1-pound chicken fillet
- ½ teaspoon keto tomato paste

Method:

1. Melt the butter in the skillet.

2. Meanwhile, slice the chicken fillet and mix it with ground paprika, ground turmeric, and keto tomato paste.

3. Put the chicken in the melted butter and roast it for 5 minutes per side.

Nutritional info per serve: Calories 195, Fat 9.1, Fiber 0.2, Carbs 0.5, Protein 26.4

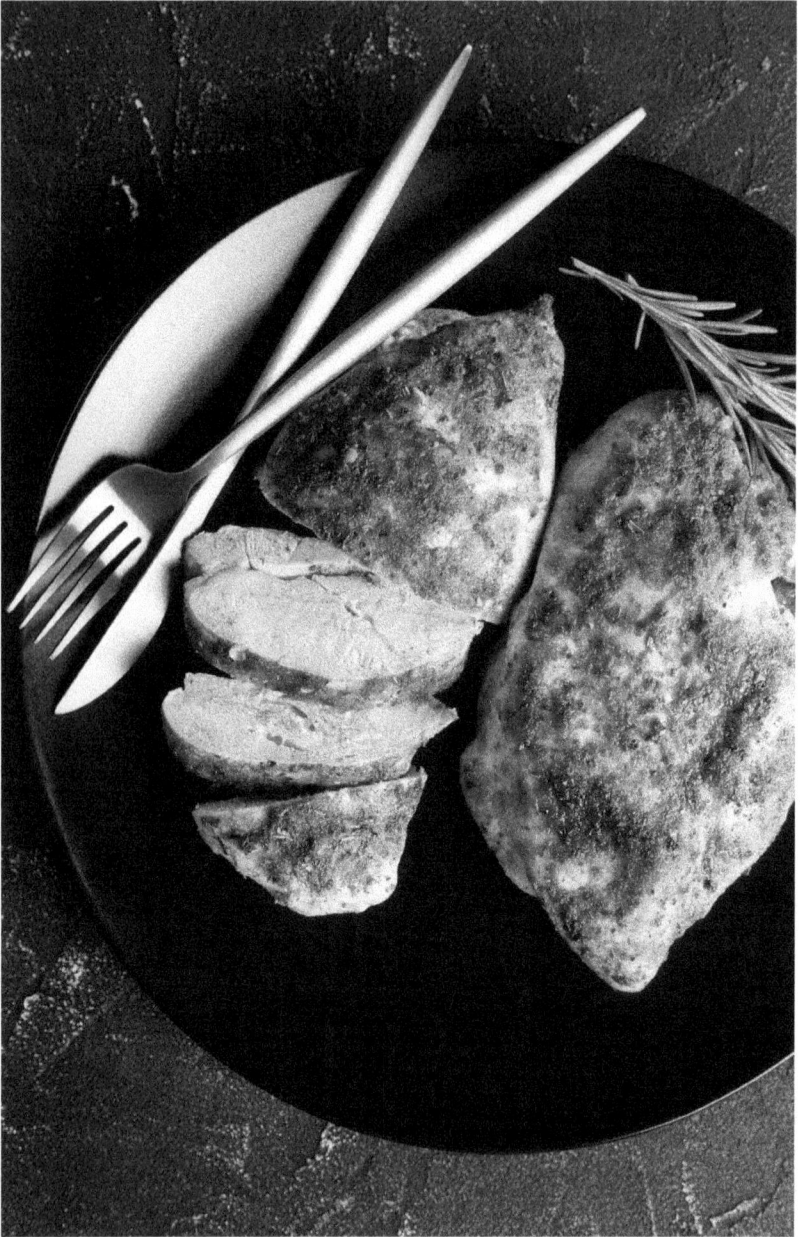

Coconut Chicken Fillets

Prep time: 10 minutes
Cook time: 20 minutes
Servings:2

Ingredients:

- 12 oz chicken fillets
- ½ cup coconut cream
- 1 teaspoon ground black pepper
- 1 tablespoon coconut flour
- 1 oz Parmesan, grated
- 1 teaspoon avocado oil

Method:

1. Mix the chicken fillets with ground black pepper and put it in the hot skillet.

2. Add avocado oil and roast the chicken for 4 minutes. Stir it well.

3. Add coconut flour and coconut cream and carefully mix the mixture.

4. Then top it with grated Parmesan and close the lid.

5. Cook the chicken for 15 minutes on low heat.

Nutritional info per serve: Calories 528, Fat 30.6, Fiber 3.2, Carbs 7.1, Protein 55.8

Chicken with Peppers

Prep time: 10 minutes

Cook time: 25 minutes

Servings: 4

Ingredients:

- 12 oz chicken fillet, chopped
- 1 cup bell pepper, roughly chopped
- 1 teaspoon keto tomato paste
- 1 tablespoon coconut oil
- ¼ cup of water
- 1 teaspoon ground black pepper

Method:

1. Mix the chicken fillet with keto tomato paste, ground black pepper, and water and put it in the saucepan.

2. Add coconut oil and bell peppers.

3. Cook the meal on medium heat for 25 minutes. Stir it from time to time.

Nutritional info per serve: Calories 203, Fat 9.8, Fiber 0.8, Carbs 2.8, Protein 25

Chicken Pie

Prep time: 15 minutes

Cook time: 45 minutes

Servings:6

Ingredients:

- 1 cup coconut flour
- 2 tablespoons butter, softened
- ½ teaspoon ground black pepper
- 1 egg, beaten
- 1 cup ground chicken
- 1 teaspoon dried dill
- 1 oz Parmesan, grated

Method:

1. In the mixing bowl, mix coconut flour with butte. Knead the dough.

2. Then put the dough in the baking pan and flatten it in the shape of the pie crust.

3. After this, mix ground black pepper with ground chicken, dill, and Parmesan.

4. Put the ground chicken over the pie crust, flatten it well.

5. Then pour the beaten egg over the ground chicken.

6. Bake the pie at 355F for 45 minutes.

Nutritional info per serve: Calories 185, Fat 10, Fiber 6.7, Carbs 11.1, Protein 12

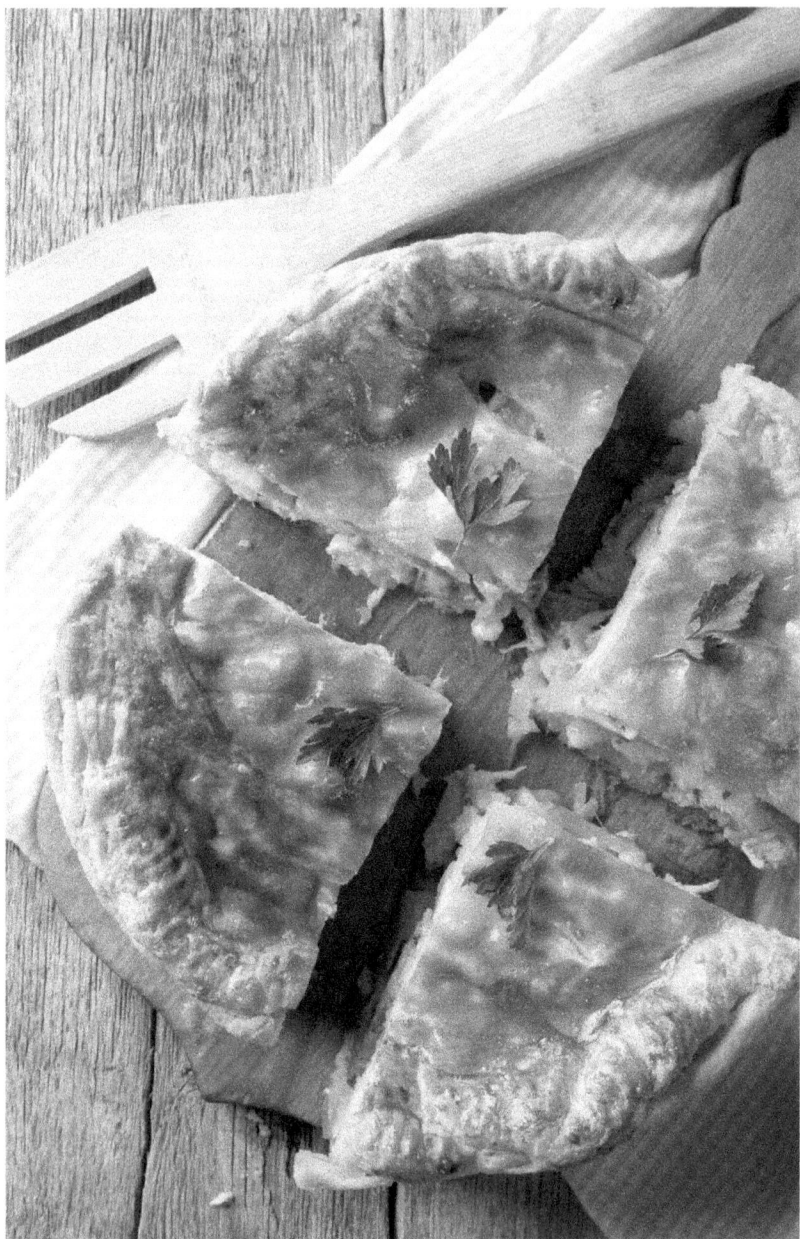

Tarragon Chicken

Prep time: 10 minutes

Cook time: 30 minutes

Servings: 4

Ingredients:

- 1-pound chicken breast, skinless, boneless, chopped
- 1 tablespoon dried tarragon
- 1 tablespoon avocado oil

Method:

1. Sprinkle the chicken with dried tarragon and avocado oil.

2. Then put the chicken in the oven and cook it for 30 minutes at 355F.

Nutritional info per serve: Calories 135, Fat 3.3, Fiber 0.2, Carbs 0.4, Protein 24.2

Masala Chicken Thighs

Prep time: 15 minutes

Cook time: 30 minutes

Servings: 3

Ingredients:

- 3 chicken thighs, boneless, skinless
- ¼ cup coconut cream
- 1 teaspoon garam masala
- ½ teaspoon dried thyme
- 1 tablespoon avocado oil

Method:

1. In the mixing bowl, mix garam masala, coconut cream, and dried thyme.

2. Then preheat the avocado oil in the saucepan and add chicken thighs.

3. Roast them for 3 minutes per side.

4. Add coconut cream mixture and close the lid.

5. Simmer the chicken thighs for 30 minutes on low heat.

Nutritional info per serve: Calories 330, Fat 16.2, Fiber 0.7, Carbs 1.5, Protein 42.8

Chicken with Olives

Prep time: 10 minutes

Cook time: 40 minutes

Servings: 2

Ingredients:

- 2 kalamata olives, pitted, sliced
- 2 chicken thighs, skinless, boneless
- 1 teaspoon chili powder
- 1 tablespoon lemon juice
- 1 tablespoon avocado oil

Method:

1. Brush the baking pan with avocado oil.

2. Then mix the chicken thighs with chili powder and lemon juice.

3. Put the chicken inside the baking pan.

4. Top the chicken with Kalamata olives and cover with foil.

5. Bake the meal at 360F for 40 minutes.

Nutritional info per serve: Calories 298, Fat 12.5, Fiber 0.9, Carbs 1.5, Protein 42.6

Cheddar Chicken Thighs

Prep time: 10 minutes

Cook time: 40 minutes

Servings:4

Ingredients:

- 4 chicken thighs, boneless, skinless
- 5 oz Cheddar cheese, shredded
- 1 tablespoon butter
- 1 teaspoon dried cilantro
- ½ teaspoon cayenne pepper

Method:

1. Mix chicken thighs with dried cilantro and cayenne pepper.

2. Put it in the baking pan.

3. Add butter and shredded cheese.

4. Bake the chicken thighs for 40 minutes at 360F.

Nutritional info per serve: Calories 446, Fat 25.5, Fiber 0.1, Carbs 0.6, Protein 51.1

Lemon Duck Breast

Prep time: 10 minutes

Cook time: 40 minutes

Servings: 4

Ingredients:

- 1-pound duck breast, skinless, boneless, chopped
- 1 lemon, sliced
- 1 tablespoon olive oil

Method:

1. Sprinkle the duck fillet with olive oil and put it in the baking pan.

2. Top it with sliced lemon and cover with foil.

3. Bake the duck breast for 40 minutes at 360F.

Nutritional info per serve: Calories 181, Fat 8.1, Fiber 0.4, Carbs 1.4, Protein 25.1

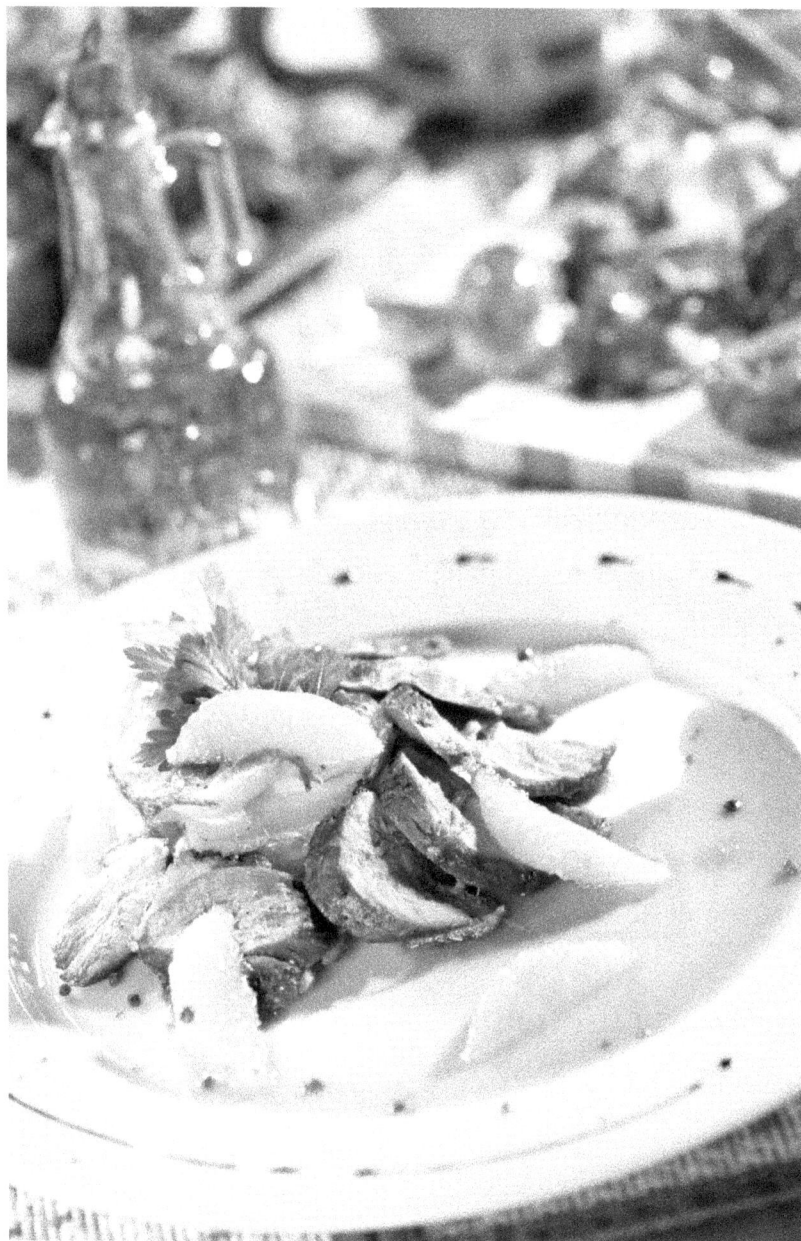

Parsley Chicken

Prep time: 10 minutes

Cook time: 12 minutes

Servings:4

Ingredients:

- 1 tablespoon dried parsley
- 1 teaspoon salt
- 1-pound chicken breast, skinless, boneless, chopped
- 1 tablespoon avocado oil

Method:

1. Mix the chicken with dried parsley, salt, and avocado oil.

2. Then put it in the preheated skillet and roast for 6 minutes per side.

Nutritional info per serve: Calories 134, Fat 3.3, Fiber 0.2, Carbs 0.3, Protein 24.1

Duck with Zucchinis

Prep time: 10 minutes

Cook time: 55 minutes

Servings: 2

Ingredients:

- 10 oz duck breast, skinless, boneless
- 1 zucchini, sliced
- 1 teaspoon ground black pepper
- 1 tablespoon avocado oil
- 1 teaspoon keto tomato paste
- 1 teaspoon cayenne pepper
- ¼ cup of water

Method:

1. Mix keto tomato paste with avocado oil, cayenne pepper, and ground black pepper. Add water and whisk well.
2. Then mix duck breast with tomato mixture and transfer in the baking pan.
3. Add zucchini and cover the baking pan with foil.
4. Bake the meal at 360F for 55 minutes.

Nutritional info per serve: Calories 216, Fat 6.9, Fiber 2, Carbs 5.4, Protein 32.8

Oregano Meatballs

Prep time: 10 minutes

Cook time: 10 minutes

Servings:6

Ingredients:

- 2 cups ground chicken
- 1 tablespoon dried oregano
- 1 teaspoon ground paprika
- 1 teaspoon garlic powder
- 1 tablespoon avocado oil

Method:

1. In the mixing bowl mix ground chicken with dried oregano, ground paprika, and garlic powder.

2. Then make the medium-size meatballs.

3. Preheat the avocado oil well.

4. Put the meatballs in the hot oil and roast for 3 minutes per side.

Nutritional info per serve: Calories 97, Fat 3.9, Fiber 0.1, Carbs 1.2, Protein 13.7

Duck Salad

Prep time: 10 minutes

Cook time: 16 minutes

Servings: 4

Ingredients:

- 8 oz duck fillet
- 1 teaspoon mustard
- 1 teaspoon avocado oil
- 1 teaspoon chili powder
- 2 cups lettuce, chopped
- 2 oz Feta, crumbled
- 1 tablespoon olive oil

Method:

1. Mix the duck fillet with avocado oil and mustard and roast in the skillet for 8 minutes per side.

2. Then slice the duck fillet and put it in the salad bowl.

3. Add chili powder, lettuce, and olive oil.

4. Shake the salad well and top with crumbled feta.

Nutritional info per serve: Calories 149, Fat 7.4, Fiber 0.6, Carbs 2.1, Protein 19.2

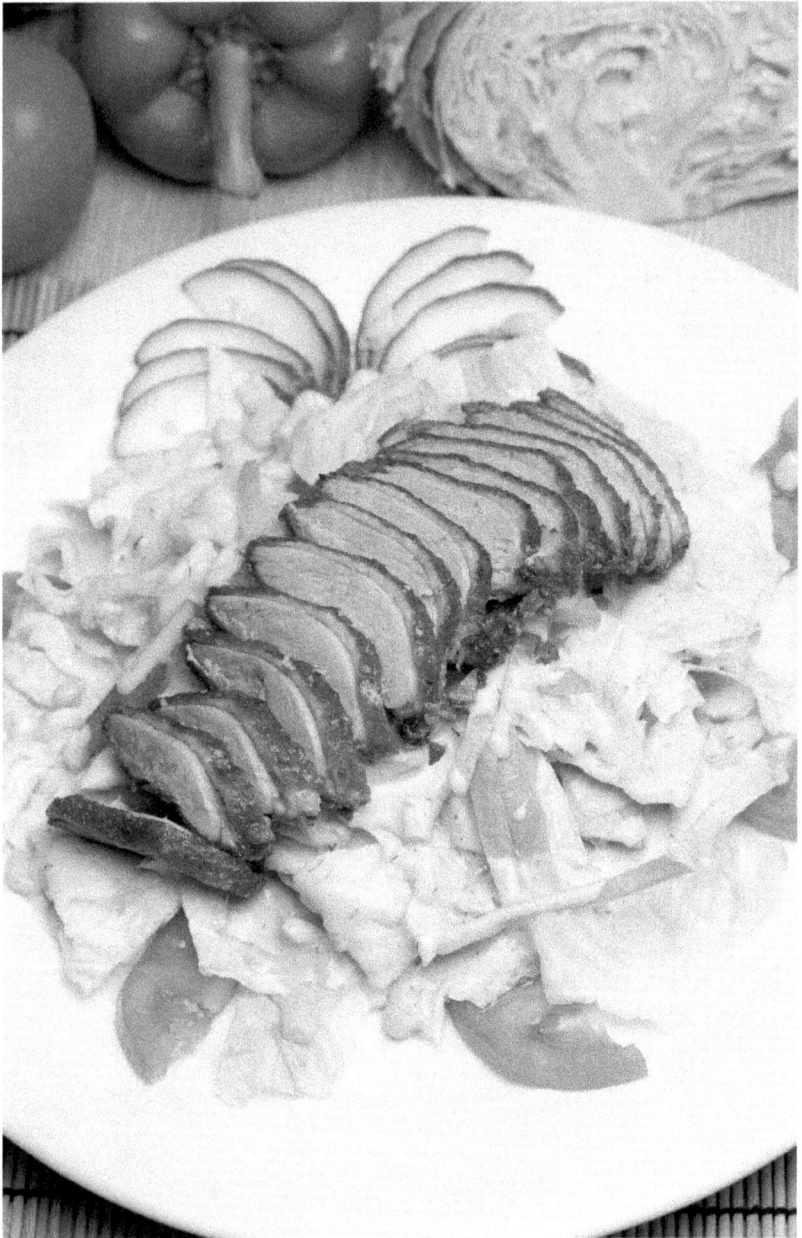

Clove Chicken

Prep time: 10 minutes

Cook time: 20 minutes

Servings:4

Ingredients:

- 4 chicken thighs, skinless, boneless
- 1 teaspoon ground clove
- 1 tablespoon avocado oil
- ½ teaspoon ground black pepper
- 1 teaspoon cayenne pepper

Method:

1. In the shallow bowl, mix cayenne pepper, ground black pepper, and ground clove.

2. Rub the chicken thighs with the spice mixture and sprinkle with avocado oil.

3. Roast it in the preheated skillet for 10 minutes per side.

Nutritional info per serve: Calories 286, Fat 11.5, Fiber 0.5, Carbs 0.9, Protein 42.4

Turkey Bake

Prep time: 10 minutes

Cook time: 45 minutes

Servings: 6

Ingredients:

- 1-pound turkey breast, skinless, boneless, chopped
- ½ cup Cheddar cheese, shredded
- 2 zucchinis, chopped
- 1 teaspoon chili powder
- 1 teaspoon white pepper
- ½ teaspoon dried sage
- 1 tablespoon coconut oil
- 1 teaspoon avocado oil
- ½ cup coconut cream

Method:

1. Mix the turkey breast with chili powder, white pepper, dried sage, and avocado oil.

2. Then put in the baking pan and flatten well.

3. Top the turkey breast with zucchinis, avocado oil, coconut cream, and shredded cheese.

4. Bake the meal at 360F for 45 minutes.

Nutritional info per serve: Calories 196, Fat 11.7, Fiber 1.8, Carbs 7.2, Protein 16.6

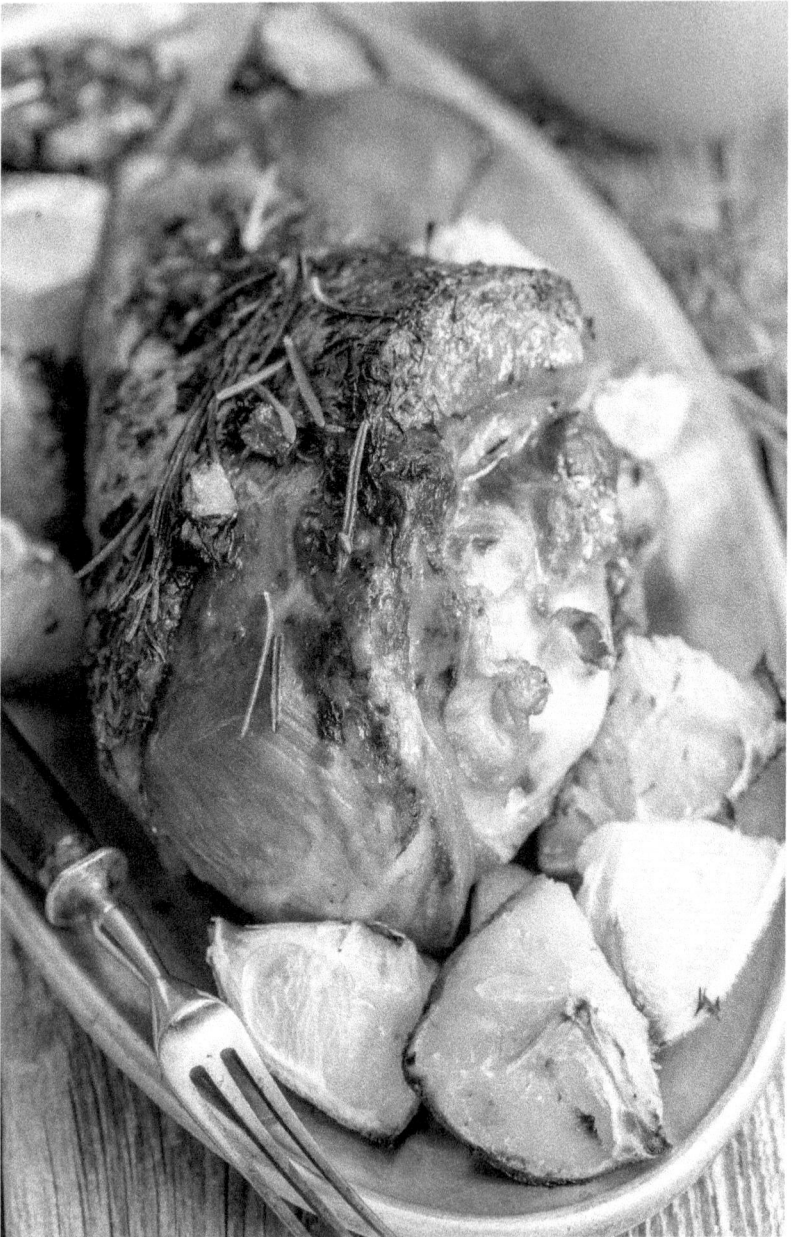

Garlic and Curry Chicken

Prep time: 10 minutes

Cook time: 30 minutes

Servings:4

Ingredients:

- 1-pound chicken breast, skinless, boneless, chopped
- 1 teaspoon curry powder
- 1 cup coconut cream
- 1 teaspoon minced garlic
- 1 tablespoon coconut oil

Method:

1. Mix curry powder with coconut cream, and minced garlic.

2. Pour the liquid in the saucepan.

3. Add chicken breast and coconut oil.

4. Close the lid and cook the chicken on medium-low heat for 30 minutes.

Nutritional info per serve: Calories 299, Fat 20.6, Fiber 1.5, Carbs 3.8, Protein 25.5

Turkey Soup

Prep time: 10 minutes

Cook time: 20 minutes

Servings: 4

Ingredients:

- 1 cup ground turkey
- ½ cup celery stalk, chopped
- 4 cups chicken broth
- 1 teaspoon ground turmeric
- 1 teaspoon dried dill
- ½ teaspoon salt

Method:

1. Bring the chicken broth to boil.

2. Add ground turkey, dill, and ground turmeric.

3. Add salt and boil the soup for 5 minutes.

4. After this, add celery stalk and bring the soup to boil. Switch off the heat.

Nutritional info per serve: Calories 110, Fat 4, Fiber 0.4, Carbs 1.8, Protein 15.2

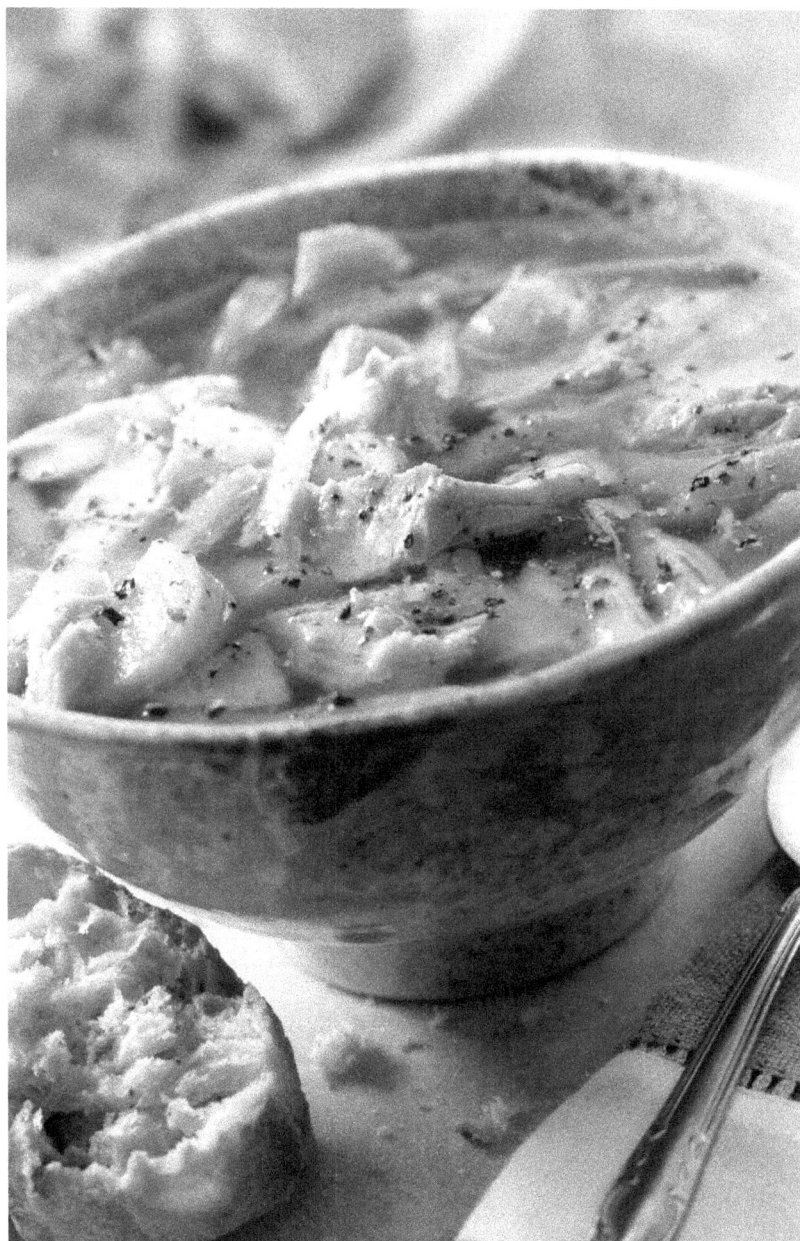

Cheese Pizza

Prep time: 10 minutes

Cook time: 25 minutes

Servings:4

Ingredients:

- 1 cup ground chicken
- 1 cup Cheddar cheese, shredded
- ½ teaspoon dried dill
- 1 teaspoon dried basil
- 1 teaspoon butter
- 2 tablespoons almond flour

Method:

1. In the mixing bowl, mix ground chicken with dried dill, basil, and almond flour.

2. Then grease the baking pan with butter and put the ground chicken inside. Flatten it in the shape of the pizza and bake at 360F for 10 minutes

3. Then top the chicken pizza crust with shredded cheese and bake at 360F for 15 minutes.

Nutritional info per serve: Calories 269, Fat 19.9, Fiber 1.5, Carbs 3.4, Protein 20.2

Creamy Turkey

Prep time: 10 minutes

Cook time: 25 minutes

Servings: 8

Ingredients:

- 1 egg, beaten
- 2-pound ground turkey
- 1 tablespoon butter
- 1 teaspoon ground black pepper
- ½ cup coconut cream
- 1 oz Mozzarella, shredded

Method:

1. Mix the ground turkey with ground black pepper and egg.

2. Then melt the butter in the saucepan. Add ground turkey mixture and cook it for 10 minutes on the medium heat. Stir it from time to time.

3. After this, add all remaining ingredients and carefully mix.

4. Close the lid and cook the turkey on medium-low heat for 10 minutes.

Nutritional info per serve: Calories 287, Fat 18.7, Fiber 0.4, Carbs 1.2, Protein 33.1

Cordon Bleu Chicken

Prep time: 15 minutes

Cook time: 30 minutes

Servings:3

Ingredients:

- 10 oz chicken fillets
- 3 ham slices
- 3 Cheddar cheese slices
- 2 eggs, beaten
- ½ cup almond flour
- 1 tablespoon olive oil

Method:

1. Cut the chicken fillet into 3 servings. Beat the chicken fillet gently.

2. Then top the chicken fillets with ham slices and cheese slices and roll into the rolls. Secure the chicken rolls if needed.

3. After this, dip the chicken rolls in the eggs and coat in the almond flour.

4. Repeat the same steps.

5. Then sprinkle the chicken rolls with olive oil and bake at 360F for 30 minutes.

Nutritional info per serve: Calories 447, Fat 28.6, Fiber 0.9, Carbs 2.7, Protein 43.7

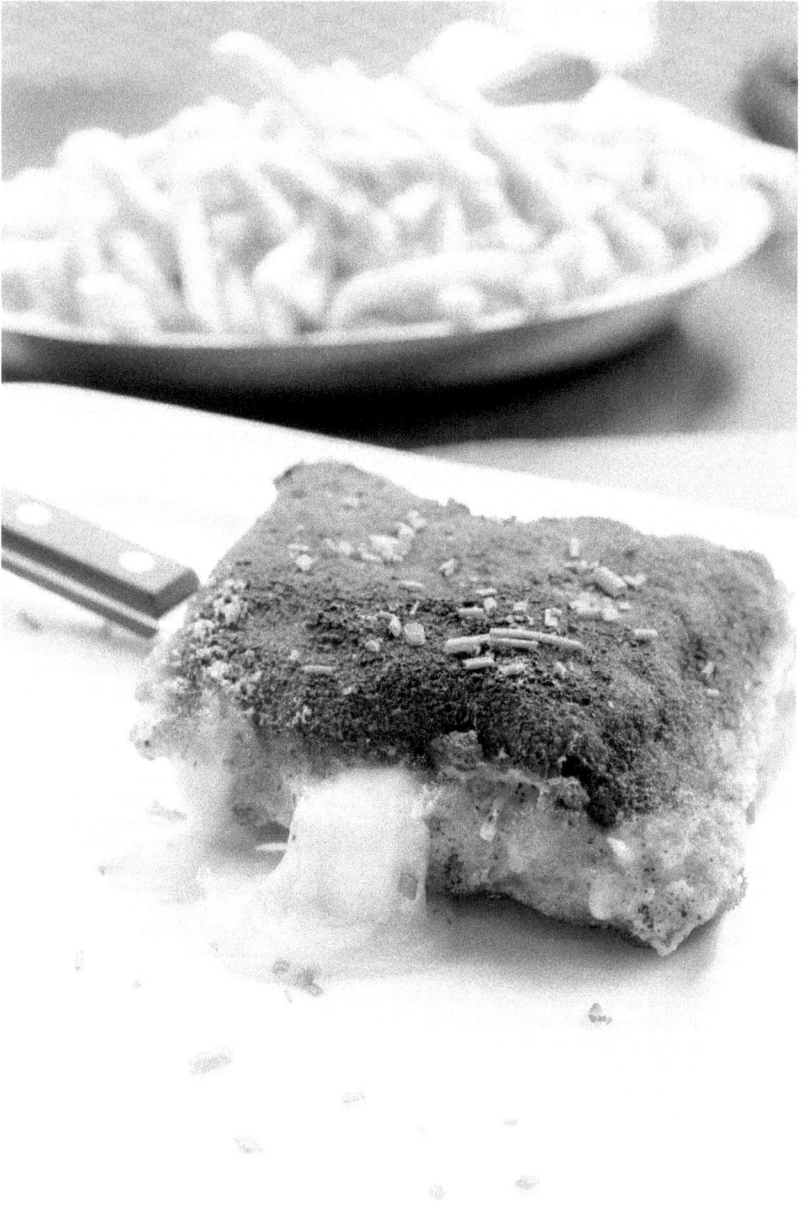

Cumin Stew

Prep time: 10 minutes

Cook time: 35 minutes

Servings: 8

Ingredients:

- 1 cup bell pepper, chopped
- 4 oz leek, chopped
- ½ cup turnip, chopped
- 1 teaspoon cumin seeds
- 1 tablespoon coconut oil
- 1-pound chicken breast, skinless, boneless, chopped
- 3 cups of water

Method:

1. Melt the coconut oil in the saucepan.

2. Add chicken and cumin seeds.

3. Roast the mixture for 10 minutes.

4. Add turnip, leek, bell pepper, and water.

5. Carefully mix the stew and simmer it for 25 minutes on medium heat.

Nutritional info per serve: Calories 96, Fat 3.3, Fiber 0.6, Carbs 3.8, Protein 12.5

Turkey Burgers

Prep time: 10 minutes

Cook time: 20 minutes

Servings:4

Ingredients:

- 1 cup ground turkey
- 1 ½ tablespoon dried dill
- ½ teaspoon salt
- 1 tablespoon coconut flour
- 1 tablespoon avocado oil
- ½ teaspoon chili powder

Method:

1. In the mixing bowl, mix ground turkey, dried dill, salt, coconut flour, and chili powder.

2. Make 4 burgers.

3. Then brush the baking tray with avocado oil.

4. Put the burgers in the tray and bake at 360F for 10 minutes per side.

Nutritional info per serve: Calories 185, Fat 10.1, Fiber 1.7, Carbs 3, Protein 23.4

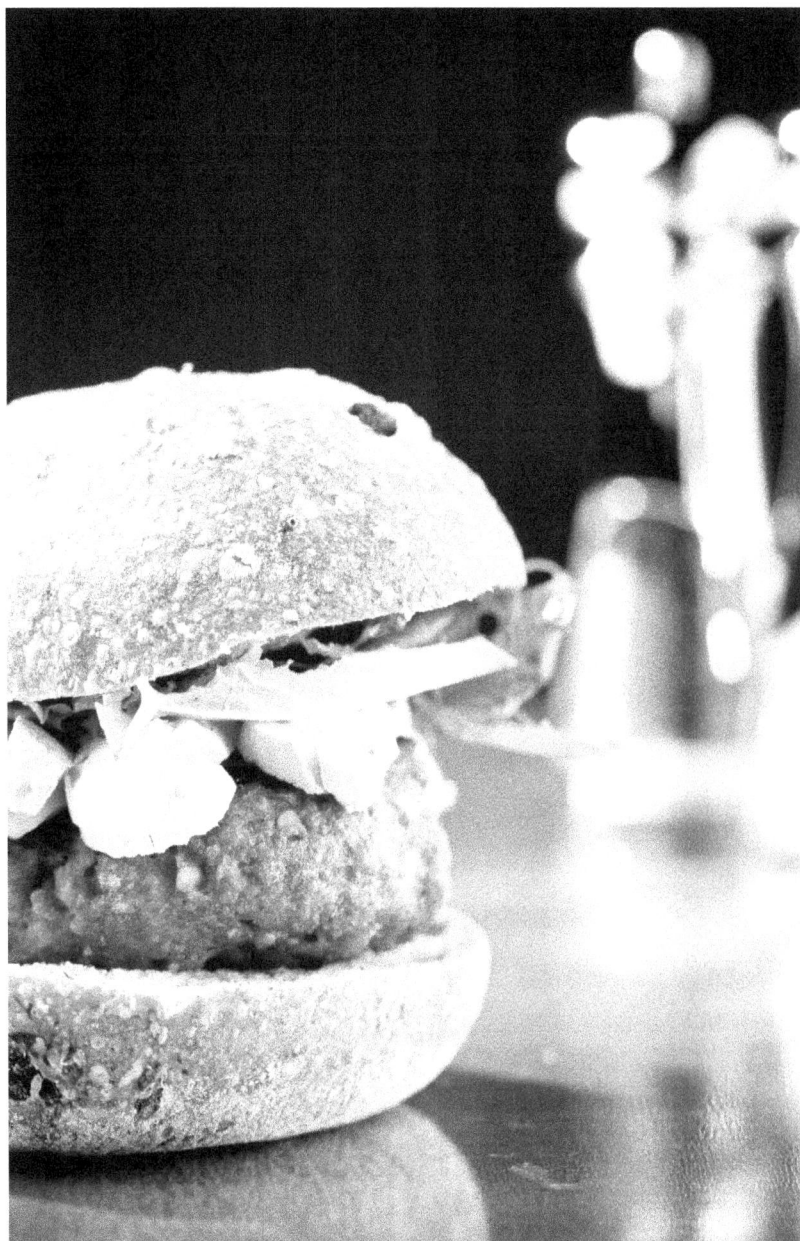

Chicken Curry

Prep time: 10 minutes

Cook time: 25 minutes

Servings: 4

Ingredients:

- 1-pound chicken breast, skinless, boneless, chopped
- 1 tablespoon curry paste
- 1 cup of coconut milk
- 1 tablespoon avocado oil
- ½ teaspoon saffron

Method:

1. Roast the chicken in the saucepan with avocado oil for 4 minutes per side.

2. Then add curry paste, coconut milk, and saffron.

3. Close the lid and simmer the meal for 10-15 minutes on medium heat.

Nutritional info per serve: Calories 297, Fat 19.8, Fiber 1.5, Carbs 4.6, Protein 25.7

Chili Chicken

Prep time: 10 minutes

Cook time: 20 minutes

Servings:3

Ingredients:

- 1-pound chicken breast, skinless, boneless
- 1 tablespoon chili powder
- 1 tablespoon ground paprika
- 1 tablespoon coconut oil
- ¼ cup of water

Method:

1. Mix the chicken breast with chili powder and ground paprika.

2. Then melt the coconut oil in the saucepan. Add chicken breast and roast it for 4 minutes per side.

3. Add water and close the lid.

4. Cook the chicken on medium heat for 10 minutes.

Nutritional info per serve: Calories 226, Fat 9, Fiber 1.7, Carbs 2.7, Protein 32.7

Turkey Salad

Prep time: 10 minutes
Cook time: 10 minutes
Servings: 4

Ingredients:

- 4 cups romaine lettuce leaves, torn
- 12 oz chicken breast, skinless, boneless, chopped
- 1 tablespoon avocado oil
- 1 teaspoon coconut oil
- 1 tablespoon apple cider vinegar
- 1 teaspoon ground black pepper
- 3 oz Feta, crumbled

Method:

1. Put the chicken in the skillet. Add coconut oil and ground black pepper.
2. Roast it for 10 minutes on the medium heat. Stir it from time to time.
3. Then mix lettuce with feta in the salad bowl.
4. Add apple cider vinegar and avocado oil. Shake the mixture and add cooked chicken.

Nutritional info per serve: Calories 177, Fat 8.3, Fiber 0.6, Carbs 3.1, Protein 21.4

Rosemary Chicken

Prep time: 10 minutes

Cook time: 65 minutes

Servings: 7

Ingredients:

- 3-pound whole chicken
- 1 tablespoon dried rosemary
- 1 teaspoon salt
- 3 tablespoons avocado oil

Method:

1. Mix avocado oil with salt and dried rosemary.

2. Then rub the chicken with rosemary mixture and wrap in the foil.

3. Bake the chicken at 365F for 65 minutes.

Nutritional info per serve: Calories 379, Fat 15.2, Fiber 0.5, Carbs 0.6, Protein 56.3

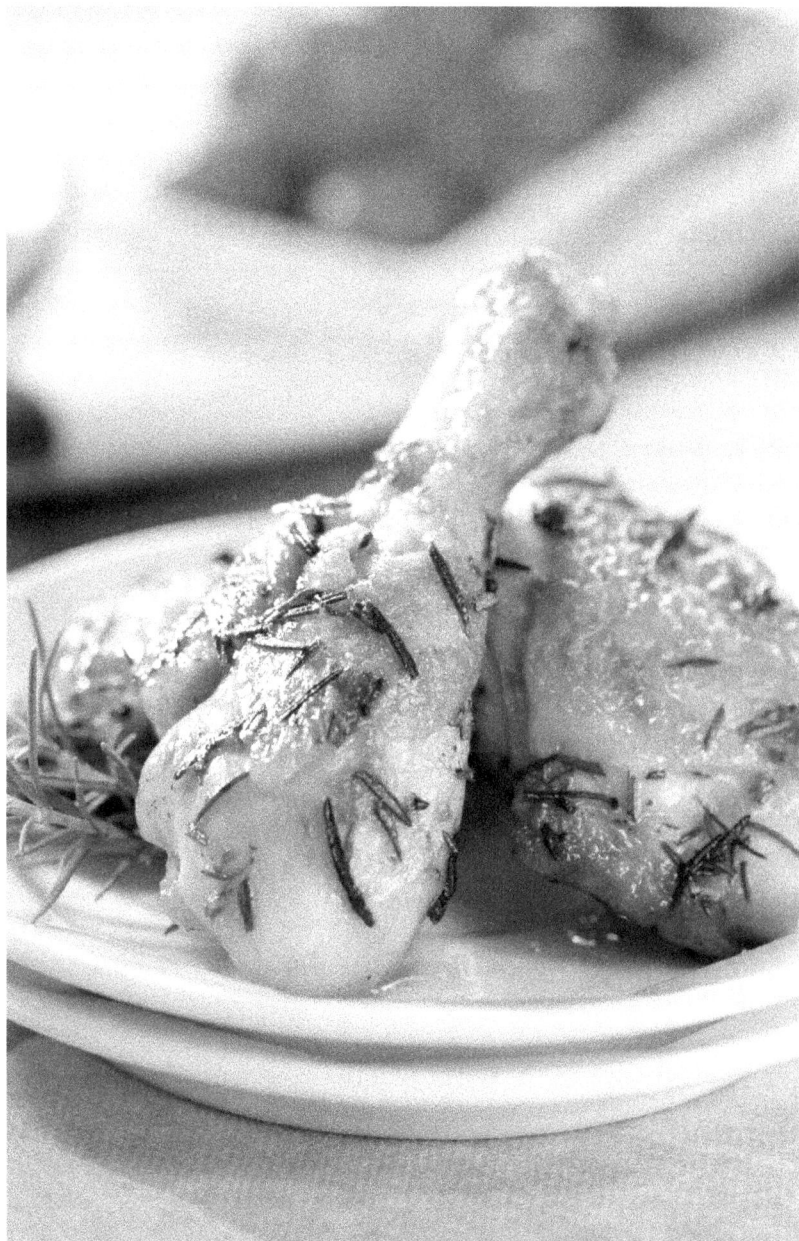

Stuffed Chicken

Prep time: 10 minutes

Cook time: 55 minutes

Servings: 3

Ingredients:

- 12 oz chicken breast, skinless, boneless
- 1 cup spinach, chopped
- 1 tablespoon cream cheese
- 1 oz Parmesan, grated
- 1 tablespoon keto tomato paste
- 1 tablespoon avocado oil
- ½ teaspoon cayenne pepper

Method:

1. Make the lengthwise cut in the chicken breast to get the pocket.

2. Then mix spinach with cream cheese, Parmesan, and cayenne pepper.

3. Fill the chicken breast pocket with spinach mixture. Secure the cut well.

4. Then brush the chicken with avocado oil and keto tomato paste.

5. Wrap it in the foil and bake at 360F for 55 minutes.

Nutritional info per serve: Calories 185, Fat 6.7, Fiber 0.7, Carbs 2.2, Protein 28

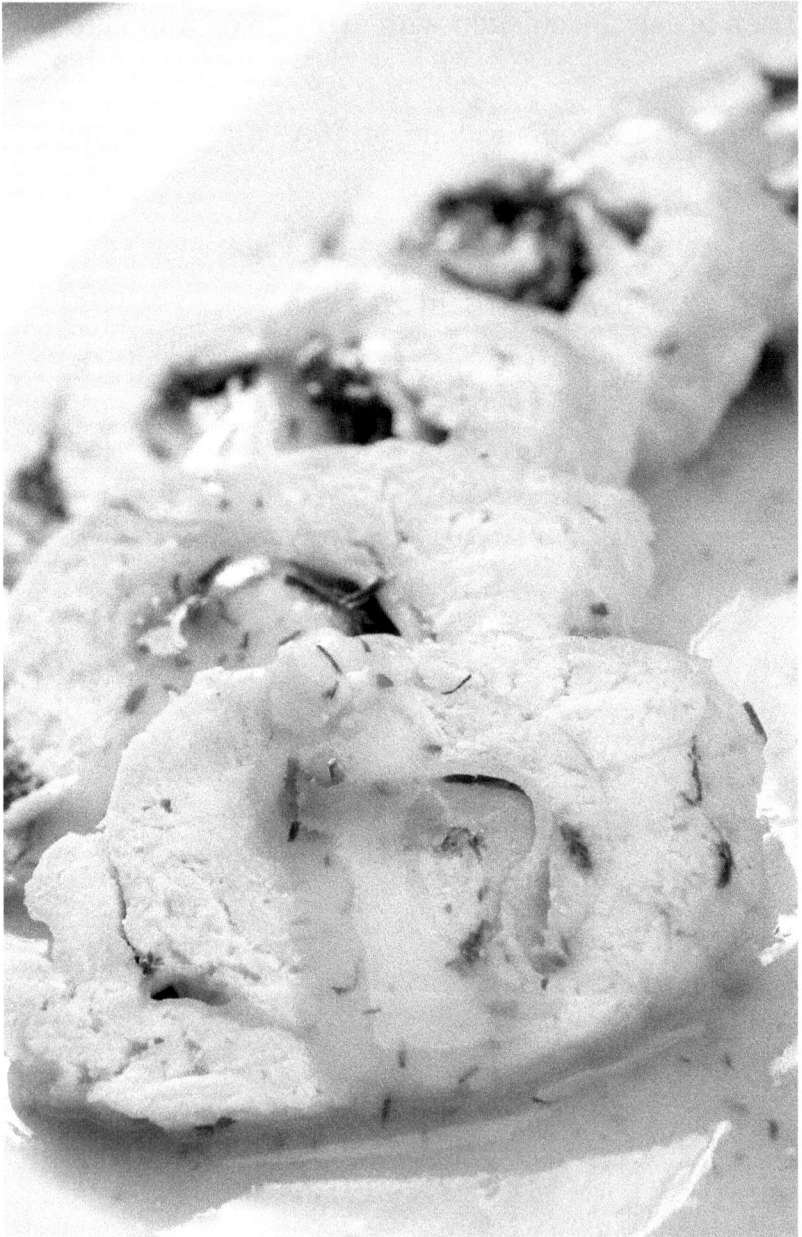

Chicken Tortillas

Prep time: 15 minutes

Cook time: 0 minutes

Servings:4

Ingredients:

- 4 keto tortillas
- 10 oz chicken fillet, boiled, shredded
- 1 tablespoon cream cheese
- ½ teaspoon minced garlic
- 1 teaspoon dried dill
- 1 teaspoon lemon juice

Method:

1. Mix the chicken with cream cheese, minced garlic, dried dill, and lemon juice.

2. Then put the chicken mixture over the keto tortillas and fold them.

Nutritional info per serve: Calories 295, Fat 14.2, Fiber 4.1, Carbs 8.4, Protein 32.8

Dijon Chicken

Prep time: 10 minutes

Cook time: 16 minutes

Servings: 3

Ingredients:

- 1-pound chicken fillet
- 2 tablespoons Dijon mustard
- 1 tablespoon avocado oil
- 1 tablespoon lemon juice
- 1 teaspoon lemon zest, grated

Method:

1. In the mixing bowl, mix Dijon mustard with avocado oil, lemon juice, and lemon zest.
2. Then rub the chicken fillets with mustard mixture.
3. Preheat the skillet well.
4. Put the chicken fillet inside and roast it on medium heat for 8 minutes per side.

Nutritional info per serve: Calories 302, Fat 12.3, Fiber 0.6, Carbs 1.1, Protein 44.3

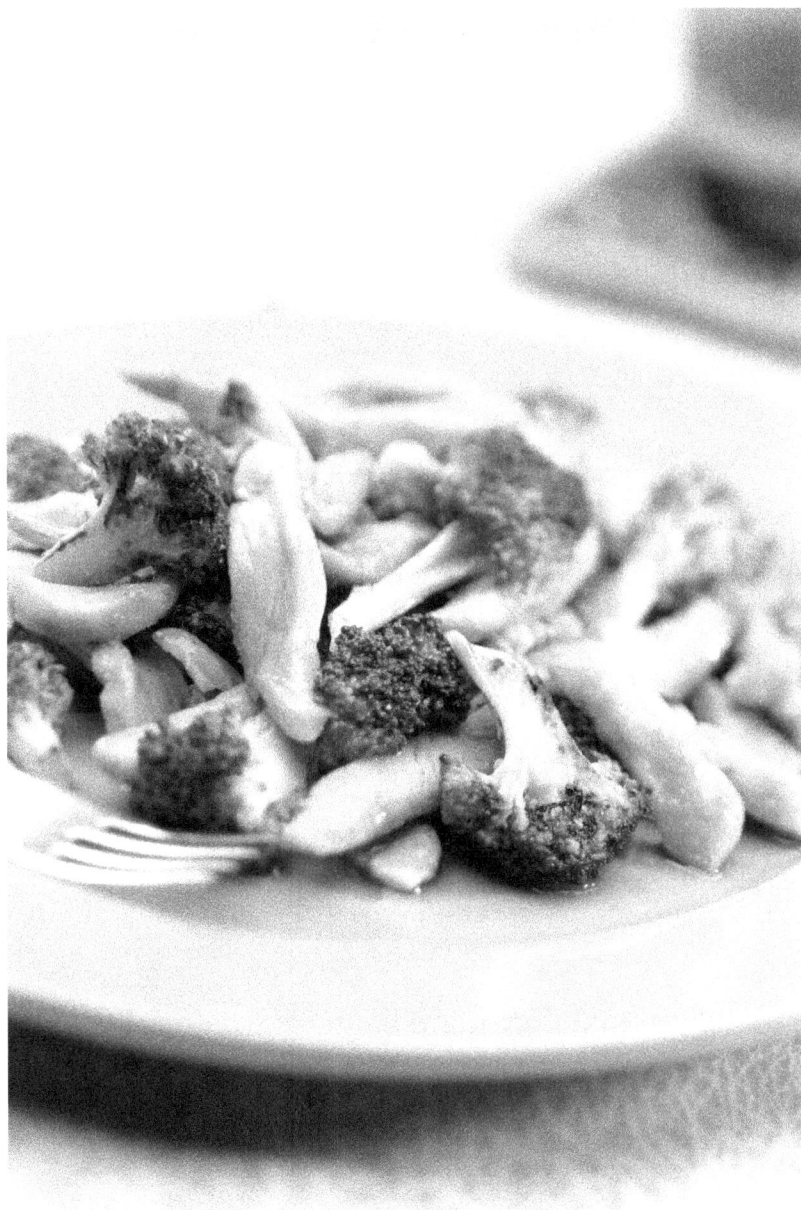

Chicken and Cream

Prep time: 10 minutes

Cook time: 30 minutes

Servings:2

Ingredients:

- 8 oz chicken fillet
- 1 teaspoon butter
- 1 tablespoon cream cheese
- ¼ cup heavy cream
- 1 teaspoon ground black pepper
- 1 teaspoon salt

Method:

1. Chop the chicken fillet roughly and put it in the saucepan.

2. Add all remaining ingredients and carefully mix the mixture.

3. Close the lid and cook the meal on medium-low heat for 30 minutes.

Nutritional info per serve: Calories 294, Fat 16, Fiber 0.3, Carbs 1.5, Protein 34.3

Arugula Chicken

Prep time: 10 minutes
Cook time: 16 minutes
Servings: 6

Ingredients:

- 10 oz chicken fillet
- 1 teaspoon coconut oil
- 1 teaspoon lemon juice
- ½ teaspoon lime zest, grated
- 1 teaspoon chili powder
- 3 cups arugula, chopped
- 1 oz Parmesan, shaved
- 1 tablespoon avocado oil

Method:

1. Mix the chicken fillet with chili powder and put it in the skillet.

2. Add avocado oil and roast it for 8 minutes per side.

3. Then slice the chicken and put it in the big bowl.

4. Add all remaining ingredients and carefully mix the mixture.

Nutritional info per serve: Calories 119, Fat 5.7, Fiber 0.4, Carbs 1, Protein 15.5

Cheese Wrapped Chicken Wings

Prep time: 10 minutes

Cook time: 20 minutes

Servings:5

Ingredients:

- 5 chicken wings, skinless
- 5 Cheddar cheese slices
- 1 teaspoon ground black pepper
- ½ teaspoon salt
- 2 tablespoons coconut oil

Method:

1. Mix the chicken wings with ground black pepper and salt.

2. Then melt the coconut oil in the skillet. Add chicken wings and roast them for 5 minutes per side.

3. After this, cool the chicken wings till room temperature and wrap in the cheese.

4. Bake the chicken at 360F for 10 minutes more.

Nutritional info per serve: Calories 320, Fat 25.4, Fiber 0.3, Carbs 6, Protein 16.8

Grilled Chicken Sausages

Prep time: 10 minutes

Cook time: 10 minutes

Servings: 6

Ingredients:

- 2-pounds chicken sausages
- 1 tablespoon olive oil
- 1 teaspoon dried thyme

Method:

1. Preheat the grill to 400F.

2. Then sprinkle the chicken sausages with dried thyme and olive oil.

3. Grill the meal for 5 minutes per side.

Nutritional info per serve: Calories 347, Fat 24, Fiber 0.1, Carbs 12.4, Protein 20.6

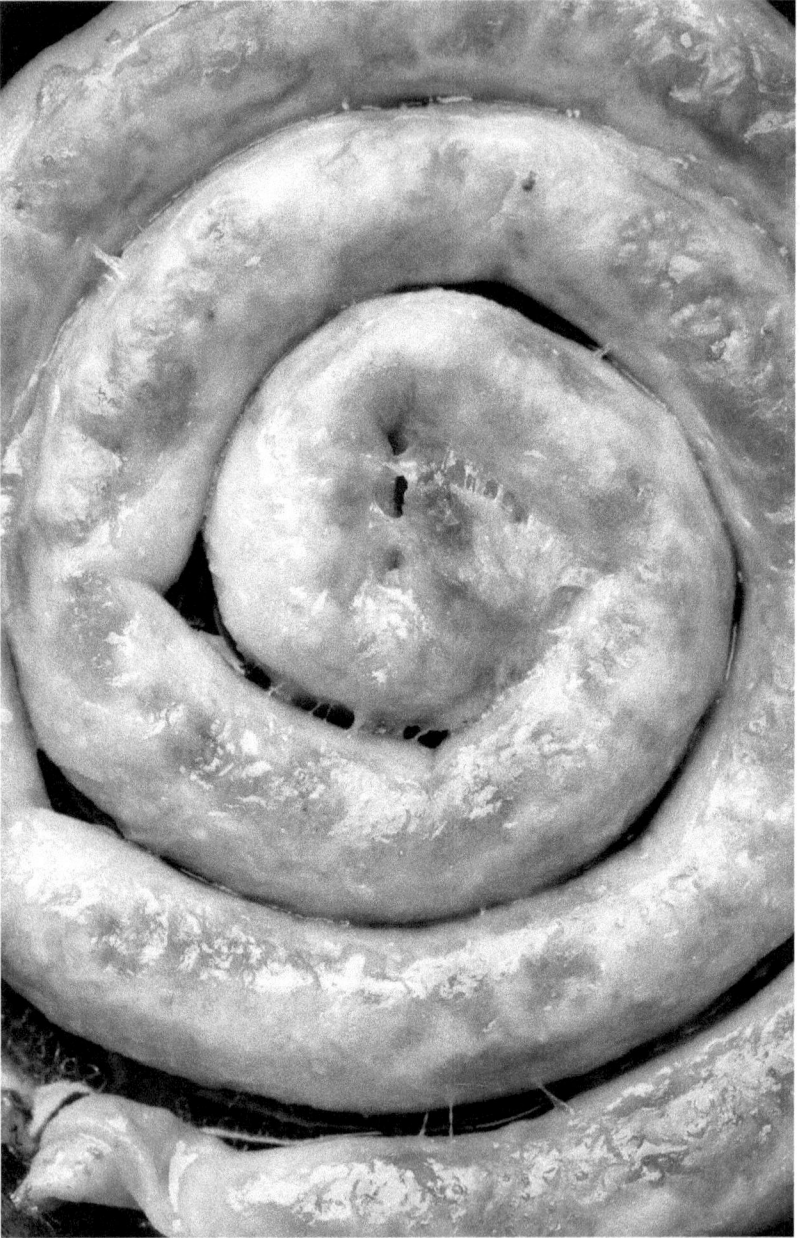

Mushroom Chicken

Prep time: 15 minutes

Cook time: 25 minutes

Servings:4

Ingredients:

- 1-pound chicken fillet
- ½ cup mushrooms, chopped
- 1 tablespoon coconut oil
- ½ cup heavy cream
- 1 teaspoon salt
- 1 teaspoon ground black pepper

Method:

1. Melt the coconut oil in the saucepan.

2. Slice the chicken fillet and put it in the coconut oil.

3. Add salt and ground black pepper.

4. Then add mushrooms and carefully mix the chicken mixture.

5. Roast it for 10 minutes on medium heat.

6. Then add all remaining ingredients and close the lid. Cook the meal on low for 15 minutes.

Nutritional info per serve: Calories 300, Fat 17.4, Fiber 0.2, Carbs 1.1, Protein 33.5

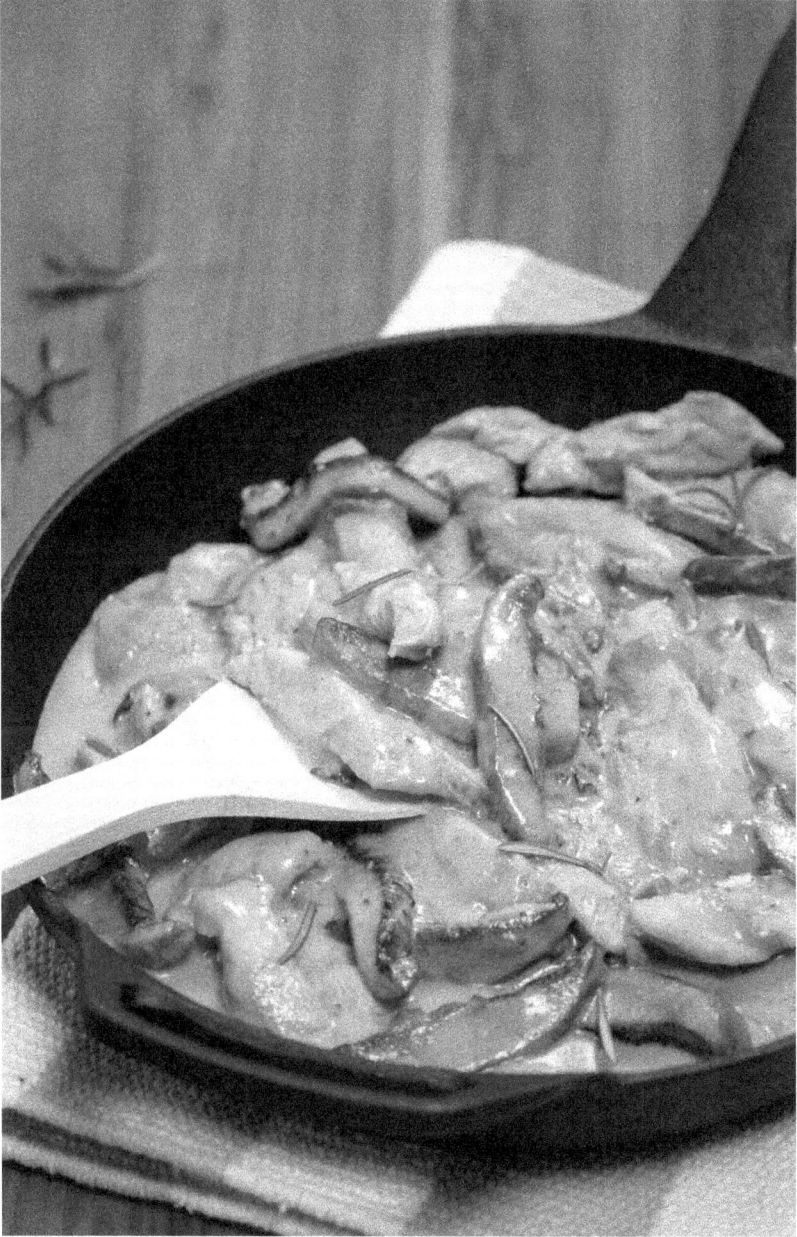

Mozzarella Chicken

Prep time: 10 minutes

Cook time: 25 minutes

Servings: 8

Ingredients:

- 2-pound chicken breast, skinless, boneless, chopped
- 1 cup mozzarella, shredded
- 1 teaspoon keto tomato paste
- 1 teaspoon lemon juice
- 1 teaspoon avocado oil
- 1 teaspoon butter, softened
- ¼ cup of water

Method:

1. In the shallow bowl, mix keto tomato paste, lemon juice, avocado oil, and butter.

2. Then mix the chopped chicken breast with tomato mixture.

3. Put it in the hot skillet and roast for 10 minutes. Stir the chicken from time to time.

4. Then add water and carefully mix.

5. Top the chicken with mozzarella and close the lid.

6. Cook the meal on medium heat for 10 minutes.

Nutritional info per serve: Calories 145, Fat 4, Fiber 0.1, Carbs 0.3, Protein 25.1

Vinegar Chicken

Prep time: 15 minutes

Cook time: 25 minutes

Servings:4

Ingredients:

- 1-pound chicken breast, skinless, boneless
- ¼ cup apple cider vinegar
- 1 teaspoon chili flakes
- 2 tablespoons olive oil

Method:

1. Mix the chicken breast with apple cider vinegar and chili flakes.

2. Leave it for 10 minutes to marinate.

3. Then preheat the olive oil in the saucepan.

4. Add chicken breast and roast it on medium-low heat for 12 minutes per side.

Nutritional info per serve: Calories 193, Fat 9.8, Fiber 0, Carbs 0.2, Protein 24.1

Fajita Chicken

Prep time: 10 minutes

Cook time: 20 minutes

Servings: 3

Ingredients:

- 3 chicken thighs, skinless, boneless
- 1 tablespoon fajita seasonings
- 2 tablespoons avocado oil

Method:

1. Preheat the avocado oil well.

2. Then rub the chicken thighs with fajita seasonings and put in the hot avocado oil.

3. Roast the chicken for 10 minutes per side.

Nutritional info per serve: Calories 257, Fat 13.1, Fiber 0, Carbs 0.2, Protein 32.1

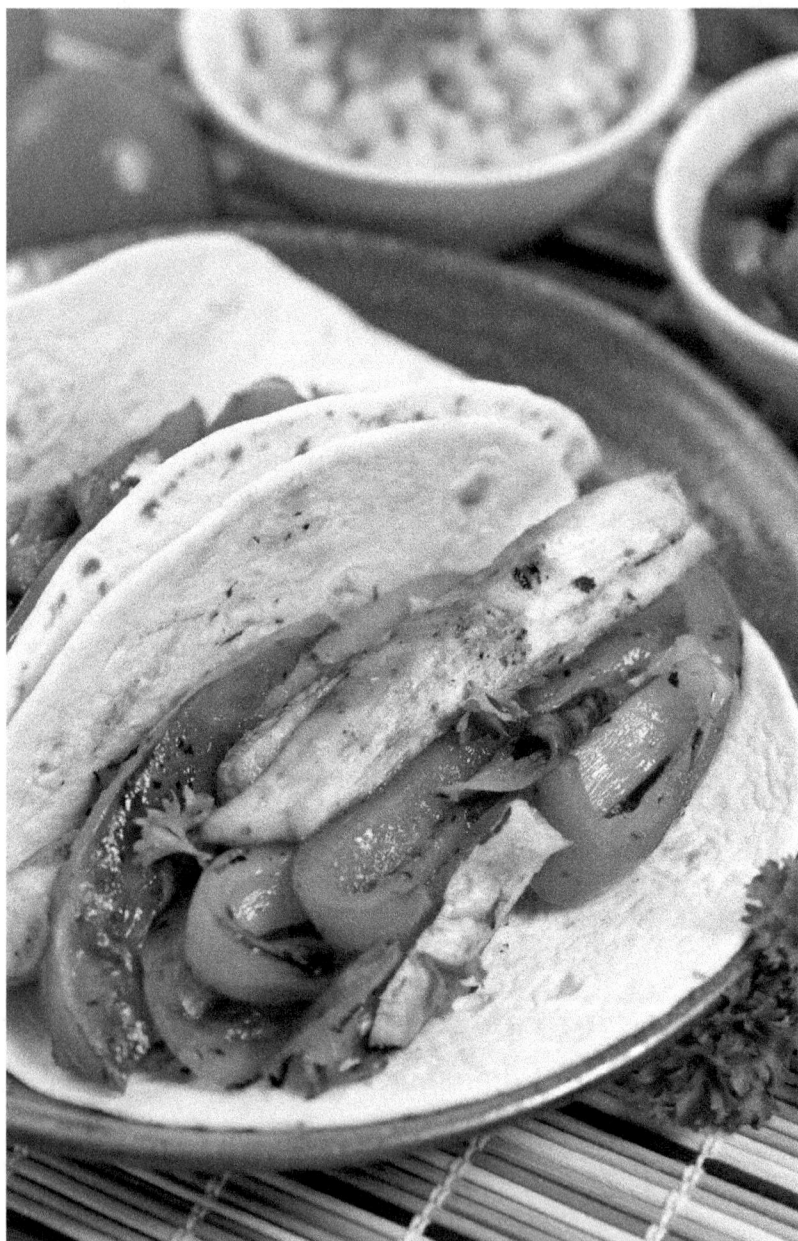

Notes